FRANCES D0578767

Ar——omatherapy During
Your Pregnancy

Index compiled by
Lyn Greenwood

SAFFRON WALDEN
THE ———— C.W. DANIEL COMPANY LIMITED

First published in Great Britain in 1997
by The C.W. Daniel Company Limited
1 Church Path, Saffron Walden
Essex, CB10 1JP, England

ISBN 0 85207 312 7

With thanks to •*OUR BABY*• magazine for their
kind permission to re-use text originally
written for their booklet *Your Guide to
Aromatherapy.*

Produced by Book Production Consultants plc
25–27 High Street, Chesterton, Cambridge CB4 1ND, England
Printed on part-recycled paper and bound in England by
St Edmundsbury Press, Bury St Edmunds, Suffolk

Contents

Dedication

FOR MY PARENTS

Acknowledgements

To the Editor Jayne Marsden and her team at
•*Our Baby*• magazine who shared most wonderfully
in the conception of these humble words.

To my chemist-husband who always pains-
takingly checks the scientific facts to which I constantly refer.

To my colleague Dr Susan Horsewood-Lee who
has endorsed this manuscript.

To Denis at the computer who has spent long
hours unravelling my script.

Preface

The inspiration to write this book came from questions asked over many years from pregnant women, midwives, nurses and other health care professionals as I lectured practised and dispensed my way through life.

It has always been a joy and privilege to share in ante-natal work, especially at such a deeply personal time. I have revelled in becoming an 'Aromatic Auntie' and then continuing with the neo-natal care.

The chapters that follow should dispel many doubts about the use of aromatherapy, and, as with all things in life, use in moderation, and with your medical practitioner's full sanction. Many years of practice and patients have contributed to the content.

To them all, I give my warmest thanks.

Frances R. Clifford
Harley Street, London.

Introduction

This clear and well-researched book introduces the reader to the philosophy of aromatherapy as a way of life in a professionally caring and sincere way.

It describes how parental awareness of the role of essential oils and massage in family health is the greatest gift to their unborn child.

Pregnancy is taken as an opportunity to focus on the role of the mother and father in caring for their own health and that of the baby. *Aromatherapy during your Pregnancy* enables us to understand how to realise our full potential as human beings, physically and spiritually, through the language of essential oils.

This book deserves to become a favourite guide to good health for the whole family.

Dr Susan M Horsewood-Lee
MB BS MRCGP
Chelsea, London

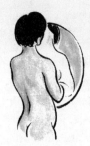

An Introductory Note on the use of Essential Oils

Our present-day understanding of aroma-therapy is inherited from the highly sophisticated Egyptian and Greek civili-sations. They excelled in all the physical aspects of health, beauty and well-being.

The spiritual and emotional aspects were nurtured through temple worship and rituals. Aromatic plants and products made from them were used to heighten meditative states and reduce stress levels.

Translated into twentieth century practices, essential oils are most often used in skin care through massage, and for emotional and spiritual health through room fragrancing, and bathing.

Pregnancy is a time when a woman's focus is not only on her face but on her whole body. As gesta-tion continues, the body adapts to its increasing burden and the abdominal skin in particular becomes very extended.

SKIN CARE THROUGH MASSAGE

Massaged gently and regularly, the skin will feel alive and silky to the touch. As it becomes more hydrated with the use of oils there is less risk of getting stretch marks which, once on the skin, seldom fade away completely. Skin health and function are particularly important at this time, and it is a perfect opportunity for the father to share in the give and take of massage. It is also an occasion for you to focus jointly on the child with your hands and essential oils.

PHYSICAL WELL-BEING THROUGH BATHS AND SHOWERS

The therapeutic benefit of a bath or shower with essential oils should never be underestimated. All essential oils have benefits for us: some more than others. Daily focused breathing exercises whilst in the bathroom will help to keep the lungs healthy and everyday infections at bay.

SPIRITUAL AND EMOTIONAL WELL-BEING THROUGH ROOM FRAGRANCING

There are many devices on the market for diffusing essential oils, but an inexpensive way is to use a light bulb ring on a table lamp, or, even more simply, put a folded tissue on a hot radiator and drop the chosen essential oils onto it.

For a total experience use the same fragrance in all the ways previously mentioned. Set aside plenty of time and indulge your body, mind and spirit.

SUMMARY

BODY MASSAGE. 1–3 drops of organic essential oil to 5ml of cold pressed carrier oil.

BATHS. 1–3 drops of organic essential oil dropped

into a pre-run bath. Sensitive and dry skins can benefit from diluting these drops into 5–10mls of carrier oil and floating them onto the water surface. However, it may make the bath slippery, so take extra care when getting in and out.

SHOWER. Essential oils used in this way are an excellent 'pick-up', and useful for people who do not have the luxury of time for a bath.

Fit the plug first, put 1–2 drops of essential oil on the bath or shower base, turn on the water, get in and consciously inhale the fragrant steam.

ROOM FRAGRANCING. 1–5 drops via your chosen method is generally more than enough for an average size room.

Essential oils may be blended, but not more than three at a time.

WARNINGS. Always begin with one drop and monitor any reactions that may occur. Pregnancy will change the sensitivity levels of the body. It is always wise to consult your medical practitioner and midwife before you embark on any kind of self-care programme. Some essential oils should not be used during pregnancy or if there are known problems with blood pressure, epilepsy or allergic syndromes.

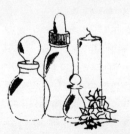

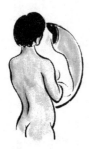

Pre-conception

Some pregnancies are unplanned and this section may not be totally relevant to all of you. However, some of the ideas may be useful for a future pregnancy. Women are conceiving later in their lives now, which can create different concerns for prospective parents. Aromatherapy treatments and essential oils used at home will work on your emotions and spirit, as well as your body. Creating and having babies is an emotional business – more so for some of you than others! Firstly establish with your medical practitioner that your sexual and general health is good. Set time aside with your partner for each other and create the right romantic atmosphere with food, flowers and fragrance. Stress of any kind (environmental, emotional, physical etc.) will disturb the balance of your bodies, but essential oils will help to restore it.

Surround yourself with as much beauty as you can – music, art, fabrics, literature, and indulge your senses in every possible way. It is said that a happy conception makes a happy baby. I do not think this is wholly true but it is certainly worth trying! Use your salary and that of your partner to have professional aromatherapy treatments. It is also important to massage each other now, because when your baby is on the way, a woman will benefit very much from her partner's hands.

It is best to avoid all drug treatment during this time and let your bodies clear of any drugs that you may have been taking. Eat simple unprocessed foods (organic if possible). Try organic wines too – they are delicious, very potent, and often a very beautiful colour. Reduce your caffeine intake and smoking as much as possible.

If you can give yourselves uninterrupted time together, 'to be': deep relaxation can then occur. Try not to let your minds rule your bodies.

ROMANTIC AND RELAXING OILS

Use any of these oils in any way previously mentioned. Rose, jasmine, neroli, sandalwood, ylang–ylang, vetivert, patchouli, mandarin, petit-grain, roman chamomile.

PREGNANT?

If you suspect that you are pregnant, stop using essential oils in the bath and in massage, especially if your gynaecological history is fragile. In rare cases, external factors such as some essential oils may cause a period to begin. However, the oils listed above are not contra-indicated.

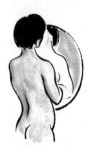 First Trimester

Once the pregnancy is confirmed, emotions are likely to surge: excitement, joy, pride and uncertainty usually dominate the list. You will have read that essential oils deal with the unseen parts of us: the emotional, spiritual and energetic aspects of our physical bodies. The first three months also have physical aspects.

EMOTIONAL FACTORS

Surges of emotions are ultimately exhausting, so it is necessary to be prepared for this and stop to rest. The adrenal glands may go into overdrive and cause a feeling of depletion which must be remedied.

A new life is beginning and it is already making demands on its mother's body.

BREAST TENDERNESS

This is most troublesome in the first two months. Try warm water compresses, or even better swab your breasts and make compresses of lavender or damask rose flower water. Make sure that your bra is giving enough support.

HIGH BACKACHE

This is usually caused by the increase of breast size. Check your posture and level of bra support. A light massage with pure vegetable oil may ease some of the ache.

LOW BACKACHE

At this stage of your pregnancy you may experience low backache from the relaxation effect that the pregnancy hormones have on all the ligaments of the pelvic joints. Gentle massage with pure vegetable oil may help to relieve this, or a very gentle source of heat.

Your partner could also be helpful by doing 'hot hand friction' (see glossary) and applying his hands with medium pressure to the painful area.

CONSTIPATION AND PILES

Avoid constipation and you may well avoid early problems with piles. Eat plenty of raw and lightly cooked fibrous vegetables, grains and pulses to help keep the bowel moving, and check that your fluid intake is sufficient. Should constipation happen, use the abdominal massage technique. If you are unlucky enough to get piles at this early stage, successful use may be made of formulas which include cypress oil (*cupressus sempervirens var stricta*), which will help to shrink the pile back. However you must see an experienced aromatherapist for help.

HEADACHES

Sometimes these are caused by hormone changes or a higher level of sensitivity in your sinuses. Do not be afraid of self-help here. With your hands in front of your face, palms towards you, use the middle finger pad all along the outer edges of your eye socket bone. Be careful to press gently at first as you might have a 'bruised' feeling, and remember to remove contact lenses!

With your hands in the same position, bring the middle finger forward to press up against the bottom edge of the cheek bone, and out to the temple. Do all the movements as many times as feels comfortable, keeping the eyes shut. Afterwards, lie down with the eye pads soaked in lavender flower water (or cold peppermint or camomile tea). Hot water compresses on the forehead area may help too.

Sinus problems can also occur if mucus-forming foods are eaten, or if you are sensitive/allergic to some foods. Consider the level of your wheat intake (gluten can be a problem), cow dairy products, refined products, processed foods and sugars. The gradual full or partial elimination of all or some of these foods can be very beneficial.

NAUSEA

This is common to many women, but generally will pass in the second trimester.

Try *smelling* peppermint oil (one drop on a tissue), or drinking peppermint tea. Ginger tea is helpful and comforting to the stomach, as is also camomile tea.

ROUND LIGAMENT PAIN

This usually occurs as a stitch in your side, and is caused by the stretching of the ligaments from which the uterus is suspended. These are attached to the abdominal wall. The stitch occurs as a ligament goes into a spasm. A gentle source of heat is the best remedy for this, e.g. the 'hot hands' technique from your partner over the spasm area, or a warm bath. Keep the area warm with a blanket.

These are simple non-aromatherapy techniques, but effective in most cases.

SALIVATION – EXCESSIVE

This is more of a nuisance than a problem in the first trimester. However, for some mothers it can aggravate nausea. Rinse the mouth out with a herb tea, flower water, or even just plain boiled water with a slice of lemon in it.

SUMMARY

Emotional Factors
Breast Tenderness
Backache High
Backache Low
Constipation
Piles
Headache
Sinusitis
Nausea

Round Ligament Pain
Salivation, Excessive

Partner Participation: Hot hand friction
   (see page 69)
Gentle massage with pure vegetable oil
   (warmed lightly if preferred)

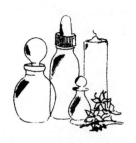

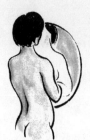

Second Trimester

Life will take on a more rosy hue as the sickness goes, breasts are less sensitive and your moods are more balanced. Your energy levels will strengthen and you will feel you've rejoined the human race! Now that the pregnancy has been medically confirmed you can, very carefully, begin to include essential oils in the bath and massage. Use the oils suggested at the end of the book, as they have been tried successfully in practice.

SHORTNESS OF BREATH

During the latter part of the second trimester and onwards, your lung space becomes more limited as the uterus expands. It will also increase the pressure on your diaphragm. Frankincense is an excellent oil to use as it helps to deepen the breathing. Use it if you have any kind of respiratory problem, and consciously do some approved deep breathing exercises with this oil, particularly in the bath.

SORE GUMS

This commonly occurs in this trimester and it is important that you seek the advice of your dentist.

However, the use of a flower water mouth-wash or herb tea is a pleasant way to clean and freshen the mouth, and keep the gums in a stable condition.

ITCHING

Generally, itching in the genital area may be associated with increased sweating, but there are no products to relieve it. Maintain a high level of hygiene using natural soaps made of almond palm or coconut oils, often imported from France. You can swab the affected area down with a flower water, and you may find that having a pad soaked in flower water gives you some relief in that area.

NASAL PROBLEMS

All the mucus membranes are susceptible to inflammation, and you may get occasional nose bleeds when you blow your nose. If this happens, particularly in a dry atmosphere, invest in a few radiator humidifiers and add your favourite essential oil to the water in them. Also try a very short, gentle steam inhalation with one drop of a favourite essential oil.

Should you have a full nose bleed, essential oils can help to speed up the blood clotting. Use lemon, geranium or *cistus ladaniferus* (a form of rock rose) as follows. Make a plug of gauze or cotton wool in a cup of iced cold water, to which you have added and swished around two drops of your chosen essential oil. Insert the plug as high up the nostril as possible, and lie down. If the nose bleeds occur often, consult your medical

16

practitioner in case there is a more serious under-lying cause.

PERINEAL PRESSURE

It is during the latter part of this trimester that you may begin to be aware of pressure in the perineum, caused by the increased weight that you now carry. Lying on your side can help to relieve the pressure, and check also that you are not constipated.

Use a lavender flower water pad against the per-ineum after you have massaged the area very gently with a carrier oil; then rest.

STRETCH MARKS AND SKIN PIGMENTATION

In spite of what is said and written, a high level of success may be obtained using essential oils and cold pressed carrier oils. The level of success depends on your genetic disposition, skin quality, diet, and how soon you get to seriously care for your expanding skin! Include any amount of cold pressed extra virgin olive oil in your diet. It will nourish inner and outer tissues very well. Stretch marks are usually found on the abdomen, breasts and thighs. It is never too late to begin an anti-stretch mark campaign, even if you just use a simple carrier oil like cold pressed jojoba.

You may also get chloasma on your face, and the *linea nigra* will darken, but these will fade after delivery. Essential oils will not help this, but jojoba can be used over these areas, too, to keep them nourished.

17

SWELLING

Your increased blood volume (up to 50%!) and the weight of your growing baby can combine to restrict your circulation. Pregnancy hormones will make you retain a small amount of fluid all over your body.

Body massage can be very helpful, and visits to an aromatherapist should be a necessity, and not a luxury. Try to get your partner to come along too, so that he can learn a few key movements and give you some home treatment in-between the professional sessions. Also, by the time the labour begins, he will then be much more confident in his ability to help you.

Patchouli, sandalwood, vetivert, lemongrass and geranium are some oils that will help with circulation and drainage problems. Use at only 1% dilution.

VARICOSE VEINS

If there is a hereditary pre-disposition to varicose veins, use maternity support tights as soon as you can. They will help to prevent varicose veins in the leg and vulva. Leg massage is not desirable over, or below, them but it is all right to massage the legs gently from above the varicosity, and up to the heart. (Make sure that you have shown the veins to your medical practitioner first.)

Cypress oil is one of the most effective oils as it helps to shrink back the vein. Use in a 1% dilution, but *stroke* the oil on, rather than massage, if you can. Use 1 to 2 drops of cypress in your bath, and take all the advice you can from your medical practitioners.

SUMMARY

Emotional Factors
Shortness of Breath
Sore Gums
Itching
Nasal Problems
Perineal Pressure
Stretch Marks and Skin Pigmentation
Swelling
Varicose Veins

Partner Participation
See an aromatherapist at work and learn a few helpful strokes!
For you and your partner: experience professional aromatherapy treatments.

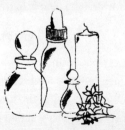

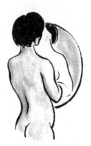

Third Trimester

The reality of your pregnancy and all it entails will hit you around the start of this trimester. It is a tremendous responsibility and you may begin to feel somewhat in awe of the whole business. Seek comfort in the fact that you are not the first, but you could be one of an increasing number of people who choose to go the natural way into childbirth using essential oils. They can of course be combined with medical care at certain points during labour and delivery.

Use your favourite oils to calm you down in any way that suits you best. Mandarin, petitgrain and neroli (orange blossom) are particularly good. Speak with your midwife and aromatherapist about oils for use in hospital and ensure that your partner is going into training as well! In this way, you can build an aromatherapy support group, which will give you strength, and help to stabilise your emotions.

BREATHING

Continue with your oils as before, and include them in breathing exercises learnt in your classes. Once the head of the baby engages, usually in the last month, you will find it easier to breathe.

BACK (LOWER)

This will certainly be feeling the pressure as delivery approaches. Your baby will grow very fast now. The 'hot hand' technique will be invaluable here, given by your partner.

CIRCULATION (VEINS, ANKLES, HAEMORRHOIDS ETC.)

Continue to monitor yourself carefully, and, with professional advice to support you, use essential oils as mentioned previously. Each week try and have a professional massage, which focuses on the areas that are giving you the most problems. They will vary from week to week, so do not be afraid to say so at each appointment. After the treatment go home and rest.

BRAXTON HICKS CONTRACTIONS

Depending on whether this is your first pregnancy or not, these uterine contractions may begin during the 7th month. The uterus is preparing for labour. If you are concerned, speak to your midwife, but you may find that you can ease the contractions with a light abdominal massage at home. Use mandarin oil, and keep the pace of the massage slow and steady.

INSOMNIA AND FATIGUE

Fatigue will often be as a result of lack of sleep and it will also affect your moods. Try to have a warm aromatic bath before retiring and ask your partner to give you some intuitive foot massage as you lie in bed dozing off. It should be given with very light pressure and include circles round the ankles. Your partner could also practice a little low back massage at some point. Certain of my mothers have found that tummy massaging the baby 'good-night' has had a calming effect on all concerned.

If you can rest and even sleep during the day, this will help you to sleep better at night. Over-tired-ness does not necessarily mean a good night's sleep! Other recommendations are not to do any exercises within 2–3 hours of going to bed, and not to eat sweet food either. The extra sugar could make your baby active at exactly the wrong time!

CRAMPS

These can get worse during this trimester and are another good reason to see an aromatherapist. Check your calcium levels, and do some recom-mended exercises to improve your circulation. Some of my patients have found that gentle yoga, or stretch and tone exercise routines, have helped greatly to reduce cramps and have also kept the body flexible for childbirth. Use any one of these essential oils in a blend of 1% for leg massage: vetivert, sandalwood, patchouli or lemongrass.

NUMBNESS IN THE FINGERS

This may be because of poor posture, or if your breasts are very large. A good full shoulder and neck massage should help to relieve the numbness with a warming and relaxing oil like rosewood.

NUMBNESS IN THE TOES

Usually this is caused by the baby pressing on the nerves in your groin. If a patient complains of this, a full leg massage is recommended, working well in to the groin area, and a full foot massage. Work also on the lower back using, once again, rosewood. Rosewood can be substituted by lavender in week 37.

As always, though, if you are concerned, see your medical practitioners.

PUBIC PAIN

This can happen in the last two months. The softening of the cartilage between the two sides of the pelvis means that the pelvis can move more freely. It is a preparation for labour! A support girdle may help, but some of my mothers have found that massage over the area has been the best solution. Use rosewood or lavender essential oil. Severe unrelieved pain should be reported at once to your medical practitioner.

VAGINAL DISCHARGE

Leucorrhea, a normal excretion during pregnancy, may increase. Check that your clothing is cotton and use unfragranced panty liners if desired.

If the discharge is a colour other than white or yellowy-cream, and has a bad odour, you may have an infection that needs medical attention.

If the discharge is white and thick, and the vulva is itchy and sore, you may have some yeast infection (*candida albicans*). It is possible to relieve this considerably with tea tree oil, rosewood, the special geraniol form of thyme (it smells like geranium), or geranium oil. The methods of use need to be discussed with an aromatherapist, but for home care make a 1% blend in jojoba and swab the area as often as possible. Leave a soaked clean swab in place. Wash the vulva area first with lavender or geranium flower water.

Candida can also be controlled by attention to your diet, and there are some excellent books available on this in the health sections of book shops.

SUMMARY

Breathing
Back (lower)
Braxton Hicks Contractions
Circulation (veins, ankles, haemorrhoids)
Insomnia and Fatigue
Cramps
Numbness
Pubic Pain
Vaginal Discharge

Partner – 'Hot Hands' Technique
Lower Back Massage
Light Intuitive Foot Massage

Some of my mothers get excited when they reach week 37, because it marks the last month of gestation, and it is from this time onwards that a baby may be delivered early and safely.

It is also from this time that I am happy to include a little lavender into home and professional care through massage, baths, etc. Lavender is the most important oil for any aromatherapist because of its many actions. You will find it helpful for insomnia and muscular joint pains. Use it in the bath (1–2 drops in milk or oil) and in 1% massage blends. Put one drop on a tissue and tuck it under your pillow to help you sleep. Do not put any essential oils neat onto your skin. It might irritate the skin and have a patchy, drying effect.

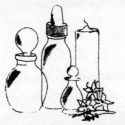

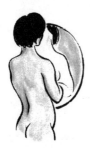

For Your Partner

Inevitably a great deal of attention will be focused on the mother right the way through the pregnancy, especially if it is a first child. You will have many emotions too: excitement, pride, wonder etc., and a deepening sense of responsibility.

The use of essential oils will help to keep you calm and relieve any stress that may build up. Use some of the oils from my recommended list: especially the pine oils, which will help to keep the adrenal glands in balance. A little frankincense blended with pine oil is very strengthening. My male patients also like rosewood and some of the exotics too. You are not limited in your choice of essential oils, and may use them in any way that you wish.

Both you and your partner need to search around for a properly qualified aromatherapist, and now is a good time to do this. A dedicated practitioner should be only too pleased to show you some suitable strokes for your partner. There are some very informative books on home massage available, and you can both learn a great deal from them.

Your greatest contribution to the baby's birth is to be there if you can, and to do anything with essential oils etc. that is needed and has been agreed to help the labour. Essential oils in the delivery suite will greatly enhance the atmosphere, and help to keep everyone calm.

Organic lavender is the keynote oil for this exciting time.

Throughout the pregnancy you will have been practising 'hands on' for the great day, with your 'hot hands' technique and various strokes on your partner's body. It will be very different for you in the delivery suite, so you need to keep a clear head, focus entirely on your pregnant partner and be prepared to adapt your technique to her needs.

FINALLY

Remind yourself to check that the essential oil kit for the delivery is in the hospital suitcase.

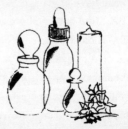

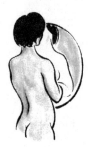 Labour and Delivery

MY SUGGESTED ESSENTIAL OIL KIT FOR
THE SUITCASE

ROOM FRAGRANCING
Light bulb ring
Box of tissues
Organic lavender oil
COMPRESSES
Thermos of iced spring water (and reserve bottles)
Thermos of ice cubes (partly crushed)
2lb pudding bowl
2 clean face flannels
10ml bottle of organic lavender oil
BODY SWAB
Box of cotton wool squares
250ml bottle of lavender flower water
BODY MASSAGE
Small bowl of glass, china or stainless steel
2 × 50ml bottles of prepared massage oil
BIRTHING POOL
Some mothers may be able to use a birthing pool for delivery. It is highly desirable to put a flower water into this to create a fragrant birth environment for the baby. Practise using flower waters in

28

the bath at home. You may need about an extra litre with you at the hospital.

HOW TO USE THE KIT DURING LABOUR

ROOM FRAGRANCING

Use the ring or tissue method as is appropriate and permitted. Keep to just the organic lavender oil. This will keep the air disinfected and everyone involved in a balanced state of mind!

COMPRESS

These are very useful for the forehead and upper chest area. The mother will get very hot as she labours, and this is a good way to keep her cool and more alert. ⅓ to ½ fill the pudding bowl with iced water and add some crushed ice. Put in 1–3 drops of organic lavender oil. Swish it all around and then rest a folded flannel on top. Let the chilled water/lavender oil mix and absorb into the flannel. Squeeze it out quickly and place on forehead and chest. Repeat as needed.

BODY SWAB

The lavender flower water on cotton wool squares can be used to wipe down your partner's body as required. You can also use it on water-dampened squares. Don't forget the ears and back of neck/top of spine (also a good place for a compress).

BODY MASSAGE

There will be times during the labour when the mother may require your hot hands technique and/or some localised massage. Have the little bowl handy, and tip in 1–2 teaspoons of your ready

29

mixed lavender body-massage oil. Get some on your hands, rub them together well and work where needed. This is when the nine months of practice will be put to the test.

TO MAKE THE LAVENDER BODY-MASSAGE OIL

Do this in advance, rather than in the delivery suite.

INGREDIENTS

2 × new 50ml brown glass bottles

100ml jojoba carrier oil (cold pressed)

60 drops organic lavender oil

2 × labels

METHOD

Put 50 ml of jojoba oil in each bottle

Put 30 drops of organic lavender oil in each bottle

Put cap firmly on each bottle

Put a written label on each bottle

The use of organic lavender oil in labour and delivery is classic, because of the relaxant effect on the mind, the good effect on the contracting muscles, a slight analgesic property and its well-recorded anti-bacterial properties, both in the air and on the skin.

However, a very few people do not like lavender, and it should not then be used. An alternative formula is given below, for you to make up as body oil with other products.

FOR NON-LOVERS OF LAVENDER!

Roman chamomile (organic) for room fragrancing and compresses.

Organic palmarosa (*cymbopogon martinii*) and

geraniol thyme (*thymus vulgaris geraniol*) for the body-massage oil.

Geranium flower water for body swabs.

TO MAKE THE ALTERNATIVE
BODY-MASSAGE OIL

INGREDIENTS

2 × 50 ml brown glass bottles

100ml jojoba carrier oil (cold pressed)

30 drops organic palmorosa essential oil

30 drops organic geraniol thyme essential oil

2 × labels

METHOD

Put 50ml of jojoba oil in each bottle

Put 15 drops of palmarosa oil in each bottle

Put 15 drops of geraniol thyme oil in each bottle

Put cap firmly on each bottle

Put a written label on each bottle

This quite different formula should only be used in labour and delivery as it is a uterine and nervous system tonic which also, like lavender, has excellent anti-bacterial properties.

HOMEWORK!

Before the big day arrives I strongly recommend that you and your partner work together and experiment with the kit. Your partner must be confident in using these methods and be sensitive to the mother's needs. She will then be familiar with how a cold compress feels and know if it is right for her in labour. The midwifery team will get on with their job and enjoy the essential oils.

ONSET OF LABOUR

By now, you will be quite familiar with a number of essential oils, and will recently have got to know lavender. It can have a very mild emmenagogue effect (i.e. bring on a period) which is why it should not be used before week 37.

If you are not a lover of lavender, I suggest organic roman camomile (*chamaemelum nobile*). This is a very sweet and light-smelling essential oil and has a somewhat euphoric effect, which may be highly appropriate! However, a strong word of warning. It is expensive and can be adulterated with a 'false camomile' from Morocco (*ormenis mixta*), which is cheaper, and has different properties.

Clary sage (*salvia sclarea*) is another essential oil for you to learn about at this stage. There is only one time when it may be used, and this will not apply to all of you. If the contractions are irregular, or the first stage of labour is unduly long and slow, take a warm bath with 5-10 drops of clary sage. Breathe in as much as you can, and swish the water around your body. Normally you would have this bath before the waters break. If they have broken, take a long aromatic shower with the clary sage, breathing in as much as you can. (The unbroken waters protect the baby from infection.) Beware of quality with clary sage. It is sometimes 'extended' with sage (*salvia officinalis*). This has neurotoxic molecules in it, which can be a serious problem.

If you like lavender, you can blend it with clary sage to suit you.

Once into the second stage, stop using the clary

sage because it might give rise to uncontrolled contractions.

EPISIOTOMY

If this is needed to help you or the baby, you must accept it. The medical team knows best. Rosehip oil (cold pressed) is excellent at helping such interventions to heal, and a little lavender can be added as well. The same applies to stitches.

CAESAREAN SECTION

This can be distressing if it is not planned, but it may be necessary for the safety of you and your child. If possible, keep the lavender or roman camomile with you as long as you can on a tissue to help keep you and your partner calm. It is major surgery, leaving a wound that may take a long time to heal.

LABOUR AND DELIVERY
YOUR BABY ARRIVES!

The third stage of labour commences with the birth of the baby, and then the presentation of the placenta.

The placenta separates from the uterus with further contractions (after pains) which are normally stimulated by the first time you hold the baby. It is very important to do this, and it may avoid a routine injection that makes the uterus contract. You may also find some lower abdominal or low back massage helpful. Once the placenta is out, the birth passage has been checked, and any stitches done, it is excellent therapy to swab down the whole of the lower body (at least!) with flower water. Do not be afraid to swab lightly over stitches etc., and even leave a clean swab in place. The flower waters are so gentle that they can be used anywhere by anyone.

You may be able to add a little flower water to your baby's first bath, or swab him/her down as well. See how it all feels at the time, but do not use any essential oils or carrier oils on your newly born baby.

REFLECTIONS

Looking back on the last 9 months as you hold your new child, you may wonder about the fortunes of other people during conception, pregnancy, labour and delivery.

A surprising number of miscarriages occur in the first trimester (12.5%–18% of confirmed pregnancies are lost then). However, the figure is very much higher in unconfirmed pregnancies (over 50%) and the reasons are manifold. You may have learnt about some of these from your preconceptual care programme.

The first time a new female patient comes to me I expect to know if she even minutely suspects that she is pregnant. We then monitor the cycle very carefully and use selected essential oils.

Without realising it, you might be using essential oils that do in fact have an emmenagogue effect, and so lose a baby. Hence, my words of caution earlier in this book.

Miscarrying later in pregnancy is very distressing, and apart from a deep sense of loss, you may feel guilty or 'oppressed' by the would-be grand-parents. It is time for you and your partner to grieve alone and have counselling if needed. Once again, aromatherapy treatments by a professional can be of tremendous benefit to you both, and the use of essential oils at home. In due time, you will feel ready to begin again. Nature's pharmacy, through the use of essential oils, is wonderful at helping to heal such deep and sensitive issues.

I have been privileged to help a number of women in these sorts of situations to become 'whole' again, conceive, and deliver a lovely child. I often use damask rose, or Moroccan rose, ben-zoin, frankincense: the more exotic or delicate oils.

Whatever the situation, if you love essential oils, and find them helpful in the positive and negative parts of your life, include them wherever you can to balance and sustain you and your family unit.

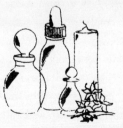

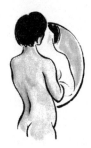

Post Partum to Neo-Natal Care

THE MOTHER

You will have cared for your breasts during pregnancy and should continue to do so during lactation. Take all the advice given to you by the midwife, but if you are hankering after some aroma, a final swab with a flower water on a wet cotton wool pad is in order. If the nipples get cracked, massage them with cold pressed rose hip oil. Cold pressed wheat germ oil (Vitamin E) is a cheaper alternative, but its rich golden colour may stain clothing and the 'bready' smell may make you feel a little nauseous.

Your perineal/rectal area will be very tender! Bruising and lesions will heal very quickly with gentle applications of a 1% blend of everlasting flower and rosehip oil. Use on a swab after visiting the wc and you can even keep a clean oil-impregnated swab against the perenial area. (Use this formula over your scar if you have had a caesarean section.) Alternatively, use any of the flower waters: lavender is best, but damask rose or geranium come a close second! If you cannot stand any pressure put some oils into a little hand spraybottle (from a chain chemist) and spray it onto the bruised area.

Constipation may be a major problem, so I recommend that you reinstate your abdominal self-massage technique, and increase the pressure as appropriate. The hospital will give you extra nutritional advice.

Baths and showers will be most welcome now but try to keep away from synthetic bubble baths! Sleep is very important, and learning to catnap will have great advantages for you. Once again, the oils will come into their own. Use your favourite sleeping oils on a tissue and for room fragrancing.

It is important to maintain your general health and well-being and try especially to protect yourself from colds and flu. Discourage infectious visitors and smoking, because the last thing a new family needs is colds and flu.

Eucalyptus (*radiata* form) is excellent at warding off viral and bacterial infections, and it blends well with lavender. Use it for yourself in any way you like.

THE BABY

The baby's skin is incredibly fragile and needs the gentlest and most natural products. Pure vegetable carrier oils can be used with more benefit than the standard non-vegetable ones on the shelf for all nappy changing procedures. After cleansing the skin with the carrier oil, swab it down with a flower water on a damp cotton wool pad. Lavender or rose are particularly effective. The risk of nappy rash is reduced with frequent nappy changes and the use of this style of product. The vegetable oils

37

nourish the skin, besides cleansing it, and the gently fragrant flower waters have a mild anti-bacterial effect.

If any of the skin becomes dry and chapped, smooth in a tiny amount of the cold-pressed rose hip oil.

New born babies need to be quiet in order to recover from their birth. A slight replication of womb-like conditions is beneficial until you, as the mother, feel that your baby is stronger. Try keeping the lights low and use wool or cotton for bedclothes and layettes. The sense of smell is dominant in a baby and room fragrancing is of benefit to you all, not only for the gentle ambience it will create, but because essential oils help to keep the air free from air-borne infections.

To help prevent respiratory infection, put one drop of lavender or *eucalyptus radiata* on a tissue and tuck it under the bottom sheet, approximately where the baby's chest is. The body heat of the baby will release the vapours, which will then be inhaled, thus cleaning and protecting the respiratory tract. More often than not babies are given anti-biotics when just weeks old for such infections, thus preventing the immune system from strengthening of its own accord. Sudden and extreme changes of temperature can cause chest problems and coughs, so keep the baby in an even temperature. The layers of natural fibre clothing will trap warm air, and the baby will keep warm in a more healthy way. Too much central heating can be very de-hydrating, and not only for babies!

It is not commonly accepted today that neo-natals need exercise, but in fact a good old-fashioned way is to take off the nappies and get the legs going. It can turn into quite a family game and become a bonding exercise for you all. Obviously you will need to find a washable sheet for the baby to lie on! Crying exercises the lungs, but listen to the kind of cry and do not let it go on for too long. Health visitors will give you all the extra advice that you need.

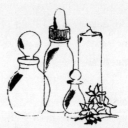

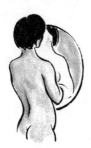

Essential Oils in Family Life

BE CAREFUL – CHECK QUALITY

The essential oil market has boomed in the last few years and been exploited for commercial profit, sometimes at the expense of the consumer. Consequently, there are all sorts of products about in shops that vary enormously in quality and therefore in benefit. If you, as new parents, want to include essential oils into your family health and well-being, I must emphasise the need for quality. Many essential oils may indeed begin their existence directly from plants and the distillation process, but they can also be extended by synthetic versions from laboratories, which are relatively cheap. Synthetic products in general can exacerbate allergies, and essential oils are no exception. For instance, some citrus oils are de-terpenated, which, in therapeutic terms, means that some of the necessary components in e.g. a drop of bergamot oil simply do not exist. What you hoped might happen therapeutically doesn't!

The quality of essential oils is a highly technical area and one of great concern to me as a consultant in the field. In my practice only essential oils correctly distilled from organically grown plants are used. I know what result to expect from their use, and use them at all times and stages in my patients' lives.

WITH OTHER TREATMENTS

Generally speaking, the stronger essential oils such as eucalyptus, rosemary, peppermint, marjoram etc. negate the use of homeopathic remedies, so it is wise to keep in touch with the professionals. If any of the family is having drug treatment, it is generally fine to use the oils for room fragrancing, baths, showers, but beyond that check with your medical practitioner and aromatherapist.

WHEN TO USE

As you become more familiar with the properties of essential oils, it is quite natural that you should want to incorporate them into your family lifestyle. If there are specific problems, it is always wise to consult with your aromatherapist and carry out the recommended treatment procedures.

SKIN PROBLEMS respond well to essential oils, but seek advice first. I have treated acne, eczema, dermatitis, psoriasis and a number of other eruptions with a high level of success. The emotional state of an individual can be reflected in the skin and that often has to be sorted out first!

ACHES AND PAINS of a general nature can be resolved with the use of certain essential oils. Arthritis, rheumatism, frozen shoulders, inflamed tendons, ligaments and sprains are also improved with their use. I often refer patients to an osteopath with whom I then work jointly on the case.

Aromatherapy treatments benefit many of us, but do not try to cut corners and 'DIY'. You could get it wrong.

WHEN NOT TO USE

Many people think that cancer, for instance, is treatable with essential oils. It is not, but there are ways to help people with cancer to enhance their quality of life. Many hospices and hospitals know a little about aromatherapy now, and will help and advise you, as appropriate.

Some of my female patients think that essential oils offer an alternative to HRT and other feminine problems. There are indeed oils that have oestrogen qualities, but there are special times and places to use them. It is skilled work for a consultant.

Extreme cases of blood pressure should not use essential oils without full professional consultation.

Epilepsy can be triggered in certain people who are predisposed to this condition. There is a particular molecule in certain oils which can act as a trigger. This is why it is so important for you and your aromatherapist to know what is inside each drop of oil.

During some long-term illnesses the use of essential oils can certainly be considered, but consult any medical professionals involved before you begin with them.

A SUMMATION

Essential oils are part of nature's vast pharmacy. Treat them with respect and keep in touch with a well qualified aromatherapist, just as you would with your medical practitioner. Babies and children are very sensitive to plant medicine, and they respond well to minute dilutions and the energetic quality of essential oils. That is why I so strongly recommend organic flower waters. They are effective and safe.

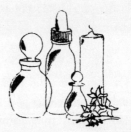

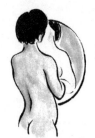

Step-by-Step Massage Sequences

MASSAGE - A GENERAL NOTE

Some short massage sequences are included in this book as it is more convenient having all the information in one source.

The pregnant woman is 'the patient', but equally well, all the strokes can be used on her partner. I have noted the adaptations for baby/child massage.

NOTE:

Have a warm room.

Have soft lighting.

Have a relaxation tape on, if you like.

Have room fragrancing!

Have different-sized pillows and cushions to support the mother and her abdomen.

Have warmed towels and a rug to keep the body covered and warm.

Work on the side of a bed, or on the floor.

Protect the back by not over-reaching and twisting.

ABDOMINAL MASSAGE

The abdomen is the 'heart' of our physical being, and is a strong energy centre. Many of my clients have benefited from learning the following simple techniques, which you will have to constantly adapt to as the baby develops! Here they are, step-by-step:

1. If you are by yourself, have your bottle of massage oil to hand and a thick towel.

2. Lie down on your back. Bend your knees, or, better still, put a pillow underneath to support the lower back.

3. Get a little oil on your hands, rub them together to make them warm, and rest them over your tummy button.

4. Slowly, and with gentle pressure, bring them up to the bottom of the front rib cage.

5. Then move both hands, going to the left, tracing out the inner hip bone, then down across the pubic bone, up on the right inner hip bone, and back to where you started.

6. Do this movement until it feels comfortable, and then begin to increase the pressure. Work into the middle of the abdomen.

7. Keep the style and direction of the movement going, and use more or less of your hand as feels good.

8. To end, bring your hands back to the centre of your abdomen and listen with your hands, keeping your attention focused there for a minute or two.

9. Cover abdomen with a thick towel and rest.

This massage can be done by your partner, positioned at your side, beginning with step 4. Have the wrists and elbows angled up the centre of your body. The massage can be given to calm down a busy baby, and be used as a way to speak to it before birth. As you get more experienced you can both massage at the same time. (Partner's hands over mother's hands.)

Generally, when not pregnant, abdominal message is an excellent technique to relieve constipation and flatulence, subject of course to the internal organs being in a good state of health.

It is also a good technique to use either on yourself or someone else if they are very nervous, or have had some kind of shock. Use it for the family teenagers before exams, interviews and driving tests! In women it is helpful when there is pain and congestion before or during menstruation.

For a baby/child, use exactly the same technique, employing the 1st–2nd joints of 2–3 fingers only. Keep the pressure very light and the flow of the massage steady. Watch the child's face in case there is colic, flatulence or inflammation. A nervous, fretful, overactive or tearful child may well benefit from this being done at bedtime.

OILS TO USE

When in the first trimester, use only jojoba and light pressure. When in 2nd-3rd trimester, use your stretch-mark oil or jojoba. For other needs get your aromatherapist to prepare something for you.

SIMPLE HAND AND FOOT MASSAGE,
STEP-BY-STEP

If it is not possible to reach the back or stomach, the extremities can be lightly massaged with a

46

general good effect. If you remember the following plan, it is easier. Have some fun and, lying top-to-toe, massage each other's feet!

Hand		Foot
Wrist	equals	Ankle
Back of Hand	equals	Top of Foot
Fingers	equals	Toes
Palm	equals	Sole

The following steps are for a foot, using downwards movements, and generally progressing to the toes.

1. Take a tiny amount of massage oil, rub it in your hands, and then smooth it gently round the ankle and stroke it down to the toes.

2. Hold foot in your warm hands and note if it is cold, hot, sticky, swollen etc.

3. Make circles round the ankles 3–5 times with the finger pads/tips of each hand, working from the front to the back of the ankle.

4. Support the heel in a cupped hand and with the other one trace down from the ankle to the toes between the bones, beginning on the big toe and do 3–5 times.

5. Support the heel in a cupped hand, and firmly and deliberately pinch the outside edge of the foot from the back of the heel to the little toe. Do 3–5 times.

6. Take the big toe in thumb and two fingers. Gently rotate 3–5 times in each direction. Lightly do a 'pull and twist' movement up each toe to its

tip. Be sensitive to any painful areas and move slowly watching your partner's face. Do this movement ending with the little toe.

7. Support the heel in cupped hand, and with a lightly formed fist from the other hand, make circular movements in all directions on the sole of the foot, especially under the arch.

8. Do smoothing strokes down from ankle to toe tips, holding the foot once again in your hands (as for step 2). Release, and cover foot with a warmed towel.

9. When both feet are massaged, rest them on a couple of pillows to help drainage. This is a very good tip if there is water retention during the pregnancy.

10. In adapting to give a hand massage, remember to use less pressure, and less of your fingers and hand in the massage.

HANDS AND FEET MASSAGE FOR A BABY/CHILD

This is another great way to bond, along with the tummy massage. Use only your finger tips, as is appropriate, and do steps 1,2,3,4,5,7 (use thumb pad under the foot) and 8. Do each stroke once only and use lavender oil at 0.5% dilution.

OILS TO USE

Make up your favourite mixture but, for varicose veins, water retention and puffiness, use any of the following singly, not blended: cypress, geranium, patchouli, vetivert, or lemongrass.

UPPER CHEST, SHOULDER AND FACE MASSAGE

Massage here helps to deepen the breathing and it may help the mother when she is in labour. Position yourself behind her head for these three massages.

1. Rub some oil onto the palms of your hands and lay them (finger tips touching) on the breastbone.

2. Exert a little pressure with your hands and smoothly move them across the upper chest to the side of the body. Do as many times as is needed.

3. To be more specific, try this. With the hands in the same position, use the finger tips to trace between the upper ribs as you sweep out to the side of the body. Begin under the collar bone and shift the hands down until they reach the top of the breasts.

4. Look for a 'hollow' under the collar bone and inside of the shoulder on both sides. Put your finger tips in and, pressing quite firmly, make some circular movements either way.

5. Finish with a few chest sweeps as in step 2.

SHOULDERS

1. With your partner still lying down you can extend the upper chest massage. Use your hands in any way that is comfortable for you both. Work along the top of the shoulders from the outside edge into the base of the neck.

2. Do some kneading and pulling strokes in the same direction finishing under the back of the neck.

49

3. Finish with some smooth strokes from the neck to the outside edge of the shoulder, using the whole area between your thumb and index finger to give the pressure. It is an 'L-shape' that fits nicely over the shoulder.

OILS TO USE

Anything that you both enjoy if it is for general care during pregnancy 2nd-3rd trimester. Otherwise, use those recommended under the labour and delivery chapter.

FACE MASSAGE

Here are a few ideas that can be incorporated into your increasing repertoire of strokes. The face is a sensitive area of the body, so use a feather-light touch. If contact lenses are used by the mother, remove them in case any oil gets into the inner eye and socket area. Should this happen, gently blot away any excess with dry tissues. Position yourself behind your partner's head.

1. Use thumb and finger pads to make smooth horizontal strokes out to the temples. Beginning from the middle of the forehead, start at the hairline, work down to the brow bone and come back up. Repeat.

2. As for step 1, but using finger-tip circles.

3. Relieve any sinus pressure by using index finger-tip along upper and lower eye socket bone in a pressing and rotating movement. Begin at the inner corner of eye and work to the outer corner. Repeat.

4. Do the same rotary movement from the inner to the outer edge of the cheekbone.

5. Using the backs of the fingers, rest them against your partner's cheeks and then rotate them. Let them 'travel' with this movement all over the cheek, chin, jaw and neck area. This takes a little practice, but is very effective at releasing many little muscles.

6. Put flower water eye pads over closed eyes and leave your partner to rest.

OILS TO USE

The most expensive and the exotic!

BACK MASSAGE

This may sometimes appear as a daunting prospect to your partner, so this is a greatly simplified and adapted technique. A few strokes confidently performed will do wonders for easing the aches and pains of pregnancy. Body position is the first consideration and depends on the stage of pregnancy.

POSITION A. Mother to straddle a high-backed chair and lean over the back in a comfortable position: e.g. support head on crossed arms. Adapt to: mother to sit on a low stool and adopt the same head/arm position on a table or sideboard. Place a full size pillow under/against breasts and in front of the abdomen.

POSITION B. Lying on the side of a firm bed, and working on one side of the mother's back at a time. Reverse the mother 180 degrees when that side is done, so you can then do the other side. This is practical if one side of the bed is against a wall. In this position you will need to support the abdomen from underneath, and give your partner a head pillow. Whichever position you adopt, keep her body covered and warm as far as possible.

The strokes will either be long and straight, or circular. You may find that using one hand is enough to cover half a back. The steps below are for managing half a back at a time. Do not massage over the spine.

1. Put some chosen pre-blended massage oil into a little bowl/saucer. Dip your fingers in and rub the oil on the palms of your hands.

2. Do long strokes all the way up the back and over the shoulder. Use fairly firm pressure. Begin the stroke at the top of the buttocks and curve it over and around the shoulder blade. For more pressure use the heel of the hand only. For less pressure use the whole hand. Do 5 times.

3. Buttocks and lower back. Do full hand circles in opposite directions. Do 5 times each way.

4. Use your finger tips to trace out and work between the pelvic bones, back and sides of the rib cage and shoulder area. Do once.

5. Finish with more long strokes up the whole back which end on top of the shoulder area. Do five times.

6. Do some intuitive work here – kneading, squeezing and stroking. End with some very light and feathery downwards strokes, using your finger tips. Keep the wrists nice and loose.

ADAPT! Use a hand either side of the spine when working on the fully exposed back (Position A). The mother should rest and sleep after any massage, and be kept warm.

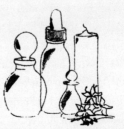

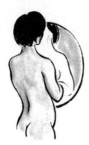

Enjoying Essential Oils

O ne of the nicest and most beneficial things about essential oils is that you need to allow leisure time into your lives.

You will also need to have a selection of the following items:

Cold pressed carrier oil.

Flower waters.

Organic essential oils.

EQUIPMENT. This is minimal, and mostly composed of items that you would have at home.

Towels – White tissues – White cotton wool pads – A glass, china or steel bowl (small) for massage oil. Labels for the 'ready-blends'.

Brown glass screw-cap bottles for making your ready-blends 25ml size (chemist). One or two 5ml medical teaspoons and 10ml plastic measure (chemist). 2 or 3 light bulb rings (gift-type shop). A selection of small pillows for use in home massage. Soda, in liquid or crystal form (for washing aromatherapy towels etc.).

BLENDING This is fun to play around with, very therapeutic for you both, and some amazing blends may be created over the nine months. Here are a few tips to begin with:

Citrus oils all blend well with each other, and some spices.

Tree oils all blend well with each other, and some herbs or exotics.

Flower oils are loveliest on their own, but some exotics will blend well with them.

Spice oils – try them with 'orangey' citrus oils.

Herb oils – good with some flower and citrus oils.

METHOD 1 BLENDING FOR THE ROOM

Use a maximum of 3 different oils at a time, to avoid becoming overwhelmed. Keep to two, if possible. Put your ring or tissue over the source of heat, and literally use one drop of each oil.

METHOD 2 BLENDING FOR THE BATH

Run your bath using mid-temperature water. Drop in 3 drops of chosen oils. Swish it all around and get in. Pre-dilute your essential oils in creamy milk or carrier oil if you have very fair and/or sensitive skin, but be careful moving in the bath in case the sides get a bit oily.

METHOD 3 BLENDING FOR THE SHOWER

Put the plug in, and drop 1-3 drops of your chosen oils onto the floor of the shower. Put on the hot water, then adjust the temperature to suit you. Step in and make a conscious effort to inhale and exhale as fully as possible for at least a minute.

METHOD 4 BLENDING FOR BODY MASSAGE

The dilution (strength) that I recommend is 1% for a mother. This equals one drop of essential oil to every 5mls of carrier oil. In a 25ml bottle you can have 5 drops of essential oil, single or blended fragrance.

METHOD 4A

For your partner, you can go up to 3% i.e. 3 drops to a 5ml spoon and 15 drops to a 25ml bottle. Keep to a low dilution for the mother in case of the onset of nausea.

METHOD 4B

For a baby/child use 0.5% i.e. 1 drop to 10ml of carrier oil and 2 drops in 20ml. If an extra drop slips out add 10ml of carrier oil to keep the strength correct.

OTHER WAYS OF USING ESSENTIAL OILS

IN A FOOT SPA – 1 or 2 drops of essential oil.

IN A FACIAL STEAMER – 1 drop only, added to the water receptacle and heated with the water.

ON A DRY TISSUE - a personal and hygienic way of using one or two drops of essential oil without it being in contact with the skin. Tuck the aromatic tissue into a shirt pocket or bra.

IN AN ELECTRIC DEVICE – for room fragrancing.

IN A BURNER. There is a risk of fire if burners are knocked over, so generally it is advisable to use one of the other methods.

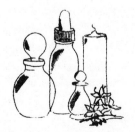

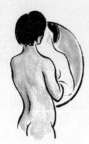

About Essential Oils

QUALITY

The essential oil market has boomed in recent years and, correspondingly, levels of product integrity have become more variable. In order for essential oils to be therapeutic they should conform to recognised standards. Certain different active molecules should be present, and the colour, density and viscosity need to be considered. Essential oils can be stretched with laboratory synthetics, or reconstructed in other ways which are not detected by the layman. It is these oils that are generally most readily available to the public. Allergic reactions can occur, and certainly the therapeutic benefit is diminished.

When purchasing essential oils for your health and well-being it is most advisable to buy them from an established specialist company. Such a company often does a mail-order service and can give a certain amount of advice to you. It is important to buy quality products as the body takes up essential oil molecules. The following explanation will demonstrate this.

ABSORPTION

Aromatherapy translates as 'fragrance therapy' and, in order to understand how it works, consider your nose. Different sorts of fragrances evoke different reactions in us, which are triggered by the brain. This is aromatherapy at work! The olfactory nerves in the nose send data about a fragrance to the brain, and a response is elicited.

Respiration begins with the nose. In an aromatherapeutical sense, the inhaled air laden with fragrant essential oil molecules passes into the lungs and through to the alveoli where the capillary network absorbs them. The blood lipids then dissolve the molecules even further as they begin their journey round the body in the circulatory system.

Whichever method of use is deployed for essential oils, ultimately the capillaries receive them. With massage there is the absorption process by the skin. The capillaries right by the innermost layer of skin take up the oils where they are then transported to work empathetically with body organs and tissues. Any oil molecules superfluous to body needs are excreted via one of the usual channels.

It is advisable not to bath or have a long hot shower after an aromatherapy massage, so that the oils are given every chance to penetrate into the subcutaneous tissue. Likewise, the use of saunas, jacuzzis and steam rooms should be avoided immediately before and after massage. If the body tissue is too hot effective absorption will be hindered.

SOME CHARACTERISTICS OF THE ESSENTIAL OIL GROUPS LISTED ON THE CHART

CITRUS OILS

This is one of the most popular groups for pregnant women. In preparation, stainless steel rollers press out the oil in the fruit rinds, the copious yield being titillating on the tongue when inhaled. Instant salivation on smelling any one of these is a good guide to product integrity! However, oils from citrus rinds are photosensitive, and should not be used if you are planning to sunbathe or visit the beach. Very fair and sensitive skins may react with minor irritation if neat drops are put in the bath, so it may be wiser to pre-dilute the bath drops and then float them into the bath.

Therapeutically speaking they can reduce anxiety and stress, tonify the digestive system (which suffers sometimes during pregnancy), and help with minor skin problems.

Petitgrain is an exception, because the oil is steam-distilled from the new growth, and does not cause photosensitization. It is particularly useful for insomnia and problems of nervous origin.

EXOTICS

These tend to be more viscous in nature and help with lymph circulation, respiration and minor non-infective skin conditions. The exotic grass oils have a lemony smell and work more positively on sluggish circulation and identifiable infections. As with the citrus oils, it may be wise to pre-dilute before adding to a bath.

FLOWERS OILS

The most wonderful and evocative fragrances come from flower oils. They are some of the most historic plants in our society's newly discovered pharmacopoeia of healing plants. Some have associations with the planets and emotions – e.g. rose with Venus, Goddess of love. It is a much-used oil during pregnancy.

Of the seven flower oils mentioned, only lavender and ylang-ylang are in a mid-price range. The others are very expensive: either because of a low oil yield, the method of extraction, or the amount of labour involved in production. The two chamomiles are totally different oils with correspondingly different properties, so be careful what you buy. Neroli can be 'stretched' with petitgrain but a knowledgeable 'nose' should detect this. Lavender oil can come from a variety of countries and species and be blended to provide a very strange mixture of molecules! Try to buy lavender which has come from a single source.

Generally flower oils help with sexual problems, balancing the central nervous system, and relieving stress-related problems.

HERB OILS

Oils distilled from herbs are generally very energetic and work in a positive way with everyday family health problems.

Clary sage deserves a special reminder. It should only be used to speed up the first stage of labour. It can be adulterated with sage oil (*salvia officinalis*), which is highly neuro-toxic. The similarity of names is unfortunate, and also the fact that they are in the same botanical family. The therapeutic properties of each are very different.

TREE OILS

These oils are very sustaining in use, and help to re-charge us. Many have a good action on the respiratory and circulatory systems, as well as relieving some skin problems. There are over five hundred species of eucalyptus, but for aromatherapy, between five and ten only are used. It is important to know which species you are buying, as the profiles are all different. There are also different species of pine and cypress, so equal care should be taken.

SPICE OILS

Many of these remind of us of Christmas, as they are used in mulled wine and other epicurean delights. They can be skin irritants so it is best to use them in room fragrancing only. Pomanders were oranges, studded with cloves, and dusted with ground cinnamon and orris (iris) root which were contained in a small silver casket on a chain and worn by wealthy members of society as they travelled the filthy and noxious streets of Tudor England. The body-heat from the solar plexus would transmit through the thin silver to warm the pomander and release aromatic aromas into the face of the wearer, thus helping to protect from airborne infection. Our twentieth century methods of room fragrancing will do the same, and benefit the whole family.

The scent from the blending of spice oils with citrus oil can be particularly evocative.

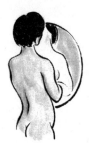

Care and Safety of Essential Oils

Essential oils are one of the many mediums of Nature's vast pharmacy. It is, however, a myth to say that because they are natural, they are safe. Many of the most potent drugs in use today are derived from the isolated active molecules in plants. Selecting the right molecule for a particular healing process is a skill that is gradually being introduced into aromatherapy education programmes, but it is still an entirely new concept. The wrong molecule may have a deleterious effect.

All oils mentioned in this book have been selected for their molecular structure and known therapeutic benefits. They have been used intensively in practice for many years with excellent results.

The following list of safety precautions should be observed at all times and applied to products of a similar nature.

1. Keep all products away from direct and indirect sources of light.

2. Keep out of the reach of children, pets, and elderly people.

3. Keep caps on bottles at all times.

4. *Never* take them internally.

5. If essential oils are accidentally swallowed, drink lots of creamy milk, eat yoghurt, cream or even drink carrier oil to dilute the essential oil in the stomach. If more than 10 drops have been ingested in an adult and 5 drops in a child, go to hospital emergency services with the bottle. OILS DO NOT DISSOLVE IN WATER. VEGETABLE OILS AND FATTY LIQUIDS ARE THE *ONLY* WAY TO BREAK THEM DOWN.

6. If pure essential oil goes into the eye, swab out with milk, or vegetable oil.

7. Label all bottles carefully.

SENSITIVITY

Some people react negatively to different odours and too many may cause nausea, headaches, hyper-activity etc. Should any reaction occur, stop using essential oils and other fragranced products for at least a week, and then re-introduce them one at a time, and monitor the effect closely.

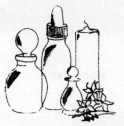

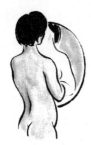

Useful Tips

ACNE

Pregnancy sometimes triggers this. Use any of the following oils in a 1% dilution from the beginning of the second trimester: bergamot, mandarin, petitgrain, palmarosa, damask rose, neroli, geranium, and rosewood in jojoba oil, as this will also help to balance sebum secretion.

ALMOND OIL

Extracted from sweet almonds. This is a fairly viscous oil which should be off-white in colour, and have a slightly sweet odour. It has a certain amount of vitamin D in it, and is therefore of some benefit. For a baby it may be better to dilute it with the much less viscous grapeseed oil.

BABY BATH

Now that flower waters are more readily available, albeit from specialised outlets and companies, I would recommend that these, rather than essential oils are put into the bath, for reasons to be explained. Use about 20ml per bath, or 10ml for a bowl. Essential oils will float on top of bath water, and if a baby happens to collect a drop on his hand and then rub his eye, the cornea may become affected. If you use essential oils in a baby bath, use only one or two drops prediluted in milk or vegetable carrier oil, floated on top of the water. The water temperature should be warm, not hot.

BATHROOM.

Liquid soda on a soft cloth will eliminate any oily ring marks from the sides of the bath and hand basin.

BIRTHING POOL.

See **Water Birth**.

BOTANICAL NOMENCLATURE

At the risk of being classed as a pedantic academic, I most strongly advise that you purchase oils with the Latin name printed on the bottle label. The mail-order companies generally achieve this very well, and it is an indication that the company has made a proper effort to inform the purchaser.

BREAST CARE

Caring for the nipple area is of major importance. Always wash before and after feeding, and dry well. If the nipples become dry and cracked some plain almond, hazelnut or jojoba oil massaged in will help to keep the tissue supple, and not affect the baby.

BREATHING

A gentle breathing exercise as follows can be done in the bath with the essential oils. Use the nose to inhale and exhale via the mouth. Breathe in, e.g. for a count of 4, and exhale for a count of 8. Build this up gradually, e.g. to inhale for a count of 10 and exhale for a count of 20. Only do what is comfortable and leaves you feeling peaceful.

CHAPPED SKIN

Often found on the baby's face in extreme weather conditions, and particularly when teething. Some plain vegetable carrier oil will help to protect the skin.

CHICKEN POX

Swab the baby down with a tepid infusion of camomile tea: two bags to a mug. This is anti-inflammatory and reduces skin irritation, besides soothing the patient.

COLIC

This should be diagnosed by a health-care professional. It is very common in babies, some of them crying regularly in the early evening. This syndrome is sometimes called three month colic as it usually stops spontaneously at 12–13 weeks. Some gripe water can be given, and/or a one finger version of the abdominal massage.

CRADLECAP

A not uncommon condition in neo-natals. Keep the baby's head lightly oiled with jojoba, and lightly comb across the scalp to remove the surface flakes.

DILUTIONS

1% = 1 drop of essential oil in 99 drops of vegetable carrier oil i.e. 1 drop to 5mls. Pharmacists have 5 and 10ml measures.

EAR-ACHE (OTITIS)

There are three forms of otitis, the most common being otitis media. Infection can spread very quickly so it is vital to act quickly, to prevent possible deafness. Warm to hot compresses can be used over the ear to draw infection to the exterior.

A tiny twist of cotton wool saturated in a warm carrier oil blend (0.5% strength) and carefully put into the ear will help with the pain and infection. However, do this only if your medical practitioner has examined the child and found that the ear drum is intact. Use tea tree, lavender (*abrialis* form) or blue German chamomile oil. Some gentle massage around the ear would be comforting for the patient.

ESSENTIAL OIL

Called 'essence' when in the aromatic sacs of the plant itself, and 'essential oil' after the extraction process. (Steam distillation, cold pressing enfleurage, solvent extraction etc.).

EXERCISE

See **Swimming** and **Yoga**.

EYE PADS

Dampen two cotton wool squares with cold/chilled water, and then semi-saturate with the chosen flower water. Lie down and tuck the eye pads into the eye socket, leaving there for as long as is convenient.

FEVERS

Use lavender or peppermint oil in cold compresses for the patient, and burn the same oils in the sick room. Add lavender flower water to tepid blanket baths. Keep the face, thorax, and front and back of neck swabbed with lavender flower water on chilled, wet cotton wool pads.

FLAKY NAILS

Twice daily massage a little wheat germ, sweet almond or rosehip oil into the nails.

FLOWER WATERS

Relatively few people know about or use these lovely products. They come only from certain plants, rich in water soluble molecules. In the distillation process, these water-friendly molecules leach into the boiling steam and stay there, separated off from the essential oil. Most commonly available are lavender, geranium, rose, sage, clary sage, rosemary and everlasting flowers, depending on the annual harvests and yields. They are a specialist product, and particularly good for the new-born child, and for sensitive areas of the body. I use them for energetic healing as well as in swabs.

FOETAL UPTAKE

As has already been mentioned, essential oils are made soluble by the lipids in body tissue and fluids which are transported by the blood. The baby shares the mother's blood supply, and it is a fact that there is a certain amount of absorption by the foetus: hence the need for very low dilutions, and the selected use of essential oils.

FOLIC ACID

Use prior to conception as well as during pregnancy on the advice of your medical practitioner. Iron levels must be good so that the blood clots efficiently, and this is particularly important in home deliveries. Floradix is a recommended preparation, available from larger pharmacies.

GINGER TEA

Cut thin diagonal slices of about one inch of fresh ginger root. Steep in a mug of boiled water for ten

68

minutes. Strain and sip as required. It will help to relieve nausea.

GRAPESEED OIL
An odourless, finely textured vegetable carrier oil. There are no therapeutic properties.

GRIPEWATER
An old-fashioned, but highly effective remedy for colic as it contains dill, which is gently anti-spasmodic and warming. Use as instructed.

HAIR RINSE
Use 20ml or so of any flower water to rub through the hair after the final rinse. Let it dry naturally on the head and hair and you will look, feel and smell good.

HAZELNUT
A rich emollient oil. Buy cold pressed from un-roasted nuts.

HERB TEAS
Some of the most useful during pregnancy are apple-cinnamon, fennel, vetivert, peppermint, lemon-ginger and chamomile.

HOT HAND FRICTION
Rub dry palms of hands together until they are hot. Rest them against painful and aching areas for a few minutes, and repeat.

INDIGESTION
Drink ginger or peppermint tea.

JOJOBA OIL
Cold pressed from a bean. The oil is light, odour-less and waxy in texture, with a generally nourish-ing effect on the skin, and a balancing action on sebum secretion. Use for any type of skin.

KETONES

These are the molecules, present in a number of essential oils, which can trigger epilepsy. However, the skin healing powers of ketones are remarkable, and they are also invaluable for helping expectoration when chesty colds are present.

LICE (HEAD)

Commonly caught in schools, but can be treated with essential oils. Consult your aromatherapist. Geranium, bergamot, palmarosa, and some forms of thyme will help to combat this problem. Use in conjunction with the standard prescribed treatments and, as a bonus, the scalp and hair will smell nice.

MEASLES

See **Chicken Pox**.

MILK

Full fat milk (or cream) can be used to dilute essential oils before putting them in the bath. This is a useful technique for those with sensitive skins.

MINERAL OIL

This is widely acclaimed for its use during nappy changing, but it does not have any therapeutic effect on the skin, which can become sore with nappy rash and lead to the baby becoming distressed.

NAPPY RASH

Frequent nappy changes will help to reduce this problem, but if it persists, smooth in a 0.5% dilution of lavender oil or swab the skin down with lavender flower water.

NAUSEA

Peppermint and ginger are going to be of the most

70

benefit. Just literally smelling peppermint oil can stop the stomach contracting. Use one drop of oil to smell on a tissue, and sip tepid tea (peppermint or ginger) as suits your taste. Some women find a slice of lemon in hot water or added to ginger tea helpful.

OIL INGESTION

Never take essential oils internally. They can have an ulcerative effect on the mucous membranes. However, should an accident occur, follow the instructions on page 63.

PERINEAL AREA

Massaging the area with sweet almond, wheat germ or other rich carrier oil will soften the tissue and help to reduce tearing during the birth.

PERSONAL POMANDER

The easiest way possible to enjoy essential oils, and use them to protect you when in crowded places: hospitals, public transport etc. Put one or two drops on a folded tissue and tuck into the front of a bra or shirt pocket. Your body heat will do the rest!

PILES

The use of cypress oil in a 2% dilution will help to reduce the irritation and shrink the protrusion. Pour some of the 2% dilution onto a cotton wool swab and tuck it in over the pile. Renew every time a motion is passed.

QUALITY AND QUANTITY.

Refer to pages 57–61.

RASHES

Generally preventable by keeping the skin washed

and dry. However, a persistent rash should clear with a 0.5% dilution of lavender oil. Refer also to **Chicken Pox** and **Measles**.

ROSEHIP OIL

Cold pressed from a special species of hip-bearing rose. It is almost odourless and the texture is like that of jojoba. However, it is one of the un-sung heroes of aromatherapy because it has a very high Gamma Linoleic Acid (GLA) content: more than three times the amount normally found in evening primrose oil. It is excellent for healing all kinds of skin problems, scars and injuries. It is an expensive alternative to wheat germ oil and should be used if you are gluten-allergic. It is possible to blend some in with another carrier oil in any proportion that you wish.

SESAME AND SUNFLOWER OIL

Always buy cold-pressed from un-roasted seeds (to avoid carcinogenic free radicals). Some shops have organic brands.

SWIMMING

Most local authorities run ante- and post-natal classes by specially trained tutors. Some of them are also midwives. More rarely, there are courses for neo-natals, which aim to teach survival techniques when in water. Aquarobics classes can also be found, given by a trained active birth teacher.

TEETHING

During this time a baby's resistance is lowered and ENT problems may well occur. Two keynote oils to use are lavender (*abrialis* form for ear-ache) and blue German chamomile. The cheek(s) will be red where the tooth is emerging and this is the area that should be very gently massaged or stroked with a 0.5% dilution of essential oil. Homeopathic teething granules are generally available and can also be very helpful.

URTICARIA

An allergic reaction with symptoms of burning and itching. Sometimes the rash is moist. If this occurs, or a rash appears changed, check it out with your medical practitioner. Blue German chamomile and lavender will help to relieve the discomfort and prevent any infection from building up.

VARICOSE VEINS

Noted on page 18, but a reminder that cypress oil helps to shrink the vein.

VEGETABLE OILS

Used to dilute the very potent essential oils of aromatherapy. Some of these have special thera-peutic properties. 'Cold-pressed' means that low level or no heat is used in the extraction process. For bulk production heat is used extensively, which produces a thin oil, diminished in colour and odour and full of the free radicals which are now accepted as being contributory factors in some forms of cancer. As our skins are porous, the potential risk is obvious. The same principle applies to oils for culinary use. Vegetable oils also completely dilute essential oils for massage etc.

WASHING MACHINES

It is safe to put a squirt of liquid soda in with clean-ing powder, in order to dissolve any residual oils on clothes and linen. It softens the water and eases out the oil. Use on a mid-temperature programme.

WATER BIRTH

A very popular method which can be adapted at home by hiring a special birthing pool. Water is heated to about 37°C and it greatly eases the labour. Within the pool, the mother can relax in the position most comfortable for her and her birthing partner. Flower water may also be added to work in tandem with any room fragrancing in the delivery suite.

WATER RETENTION

A common problem in the third trimester which can be relieved by foot and leg massage. Lemongrass, geranium or sandalwood oils are helpful, and remember to keep the legs up as much as possible.

WHEAT GERM OIL

Vitamin E oil. It is cold-pressed from wheat, is a rich golden colour and has a bread-like odour. Do not use if you are allergic to wheat (gluten). It is well known for its antioxidant and regenerative effect on damaged tissue.

YOGA

This is always beneficial during and after pregnancy, and I strongly recommend it. It can be used to relax, keep fit and supple, and also as a type of meditation. There are different types of yoga, hatha yoga being physically orientated and also involving particular attention to the breath.

YOGHURT

This is an alternative medium for diluting essential oils to float in a bath. Use the live yoghurt. It may also be applied to inflamed and infected skin.

ZINGIBER OFFICINALIS

To my ear this is a delightfully onomatopoeic term for ginger. A highly energetic oil and in other forms is much used in Eastern medical practice: in China in particular.

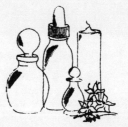

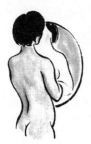

Epilogue

Lavender oil has become a very special fragrance since the birth of my son.

My husband used it to massage me during labour and we used the oil to scent the room during the birth. Whenever I smell lavender now it reminds me of our truly wonderful day.

From a recent patient.
1996.

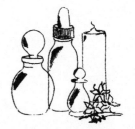

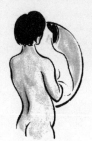

Useful Addresses

WHERE TO FIND A QUALIFIED AND INSURED AROMATHERAPIST

Aromatherapy Organisations Council
(A.O.C)
3 Latymer Close
Braybrooke
Market Harborough
Leicester LE16 8LN
Tel: 01858 434242
Send an A5 S.A.E. for a booklet, which will list training organisations and give general information on aromatherapy worldwide.

British Register of Complementary Practitioners (B.R.C.P.)
P.O.B. 194
London SE16 1QZ
Send a S.A.E. for information and practitioner contacts worldwide.

Guild of Complementary Practitioners

Liddell House
Liddell Close
Finchampstead
Berkshire
RG40 4NS
Tel: 01734-735757
Fax: 01734-735767

A professional association of qualified complementary care practitioners, and in particular, aromatherapists. The Guild has worldwide contacts.

Register of Qualified Aromatherapists

(R.Q.A.)
P.O.B. 3431
Stanbury
Chelmsford
Essex CM3 4UA
Tel: 01245 227957
Fax: 01245 222152

SECTION 2

SUPPLIERS, ASSOCIATIOINS AND SERVICES

Foresight Association

88 The Paddock
Godalming
Surrey
GU7 1XD
Tel: 01483-427839

Send 31p S.A.E. for an information pack.
A pioneering group to advise on all aspects of preconceptual care.

National Childbirth Trust
Alexandra House
Oldham Terrace
London W3 6NH
Tel: 0181-992 8637
Fax: 0181-992 9929
A long established trust offering classes and information on all aspects of child birth.
They also have a worldwide mail order service.

Splashdown Water Birth Services
17 Wellington Terrace
Harrow on the Hill
Middlesex HA1 3EP
Tel: 0181-422 9308
Birthing pools available for hire for NHS or private births worldwide. It is also a centre of education for parents to be and is English National Board approved.

Active Birth Centre
25 Bickerton Road
London N19 5JT
Tel: 0171-561 9006
Fax: 0171-561 9007
Birthing pools for hire, with water births and yoga workshops held regularly. An excellent catalogue is also available worldwide listing up to date products from books to bras. The Centre also has a small worldwide network of trained active birth teachers.

Caroline Flint Midwifery Services
The Birth Centre Ltd
34 Elm Quay Court
Nine Elms Lane
London SW8 5DE
Tel: 0171-498 2322
Fax: 0171-498 0698
An innovative birth centre providing private facili-
ties with instant access to St George's Hospital.

The Birth Unit
Hospital of St John and St Elizabeth
60 Grove End Road
London N1U8 GNH
Tel: 0171-286 5126
Fax: 0171-266 4813
A private unit established previously in the Garden
Hospital, Hendon. It is an international centre for
natural birth and the use of complementary thera-
pies during pregnancy and labour. A large midwife
team is headed up by two obstetricians.

Higher Nature Ltd
Burwash Common
East Sussex
TN19 7LX
Tel: 01435-882880 (World wide mail order)
Fax: 01435-883720
An established company which excels in the supply
of ethical supplements, and is a particularly recom-
mended supplier of Folacin (folic acid). Vegetarian
and vegan requirements are taken into consideration.

'Little Dippers'
2/4 West Street
Rottingdean
Brighton
East Sussex BN2 7HP
Tel: 01273-307155
Courses are run for Mother and Baby to develop life-saving skills in water. It will also promote strength and general health, and develop the respiratory system. Learning these skills at such a young age provides mental stimulation and most importantly a chance for early parental bonding.

Bodytreats International Ltd
(Group established in 1982)
15 Approach Road
London SW20 8BA
Tel: 0181-543 7633 (World wide mail order)
Fax: 0181-543 9600
Mobile: 0468-908486 (World wide mail order)
Mobile: 0370-790055 (Clinic)
E-mail: cliffords@bodytreats.com
Web: www.bodytreats.com
Specialist suppliers of organic oils, flower waters and vegetable carrier oils. The company is headed by a chemist and a consultant aromatherapist who work jointly together to promote health and well-being using these scientifically profiled products.

SECTION 3

ORGANIZATIONS OUTSIDE THE UK

AUSTRALIA

International Federation of Aromatherapists

P.O. Box 107,
Burwood,
N.S.W., 2904
Tel: 190 224 0125

CANADA

Alberta Society for Professional Aromatherapists

204 Queensland Place, SE,
Calgary,
Alberta,
T2J 4E2
Tel: (403) 278 9788

ISRAEL

Israeli College of Natural Health Sciences

P.O.B. 29627,
Tel Aviv, 61296
Tel: 3 6888838

JAPAN

International Federation of Aromatherapists

2-8-3-706 Shibaura,
Minato-ku,
Tokyo, 108
Tel: 813 3769 0935

New Zealand Register of Holistic Aromatherapists
PO Box 18-399,
Glenn Innes,
Auckland 6,
New Zealand
Tel: St Heliers 575 6636

Association of Aromatherapists Southern Africa
PO Box 23924,
Claremont 7735,
Republic of South Africa
Tel: 021 5312979/021 7943660
Fax: 021 7947298

Morris Institute of Natural Therapeutics
3108 Route 10 West,
Denville,
New Jersey, 07834,
U.S.A.
Tel: (201) 989 8939

National Association for Holistic Aromatherapy
219 Carl Street,
San Francisco,
CA 94117,
U.S.A.
Tel: (415) 564 6785
Fax: (415) 564 6799

Essential Oil Chart – Citrus

Essential Oil	Botanical name	Part of plant used	Method of use	Female massage Trimester			Male massage	Baby baths & massage	Main use in the family
				1	2	3			
Bergamot	Citrus Bergamia	Rind	1.2.3.4	✗	✓	✓	✓	✗	Nervous depression, sedative, insomnia, anti-bacterial
Bitter Orange	Citrus Aurantium	Rind	1.2.3.4	✗	✓	✓	✓	✗	Anxiety, sedative, gastric spasm, flatulence
Grapefruit	Citrus Paradisii	Rind	1.2.3.4	✗	✗	✗	✗	✗	Air freshener
Lemon	Citrus Limonum	Rind	1.2.3.4	✗	✓	✓	✓	✗	Anti-viral, hyperactivity, slow circulation
Lime	Citrus Limetta	Rind	1. 3	✗	✗	✗	✗	✗	Air freshener
Mandarin	Citrus Reticulata	Rind	1.2.3.4	✗	✓	✓	✓	✗	Sedative, digestive tonic, anti-fungal
Petitgrain	Citrus Aurantium	Leaves/Flower Buds	1.2.3.4	✗	✓	✓	✓	✗	Insomnia, muscular cramps of nervous origin, flatulence, antibacterial
Sweet Orange	Citrus Sinensis	Rind	1.2.3.4	✗	✓	✓	✓	✗	Sedative, helps digestion

Essential Oil Chart

Essential Oil Chart – Exotics

Essential Oil	Botanical name	Part of plant used	Method of use	Female massage Trimester			Male massage	Baby baths & massage	Main use in the family
				1	2	3			
Benzoin	Styrax Benzoe	Resin	1.2.3.4	✗	✓	✓	✓	✗	Use for all skin problems, relaxing
Frankincense	Boswellia Carterii	Resin	1.2.3.4	✗	✓	✓	✓	✗	Deepens breathing, boosts immune system, skinhealing
Lemongrass	Cymbopogon Citratus	Grass-leaves	1.2.3.4	✗	✓	✓	✓	✗	Sedative. Aids leg circulation
Palmarosa	Cymbopogon Martinii	Grass-leaves	1.2.3.4	✗	✗	✓	✓	✗	Anti-fungal, labour, certain eczemas, anti-viral, sinusitis, bronchitis, cystitis
Patchouli	Pogostemon Cablin	Leaves	1.2.3.4	✗	✓	✓	✓	✗	Skin problems, swollen legs and feet, piles, relaxing, aphrodisiac
Vetivert	Vetiveria Zizanoides	Roots	1.2.3.4	✗	✓	✓	✓	✗	Maintains health of lymph, relaxing, aphrodisiac, urticaria

85

Essential Oil Chart – Flowers

Essential Oil	Botanical name	Part of plant used	Method of use	Female massage Trimester 1	2	3	Male massage	Baby baths & massage	Main use in the family
Blue Chamomile	Matricaria Recutita	Flowers	1.2.3	✗	✗	✗	✓	✓	Cystitis, inflammatory skin problems
Damask Rose	Rosa Damascena	Petals	1.2.3.4	✗	✓	✓	✓	✓	Nervous fatigue, sexual exhaustion, frigidity, impotence, skin problems, gingivitis
Jasmine	Jasminium Grandiflora	Flowers	1.2.3.4	✗	✗	✓	✓	✗	Sexual exhaustion, impotence, frigidity, insomnia
Lavender	Lavandula Angustifolia	Flowers	1.2.3.4	✗	✓	✓	✓	✓	Anti-viral, anti-bacterial, labour, skin healing, muscular cramps
Neroli	Citrus Aurantium	Flowers	1.2.3.4	✗	✓	✓	✓	✓	Nervous fatigue, diarrhoea, digestive tonic, skin care, leg tension, insomnia
Roman Chamomile	Chamaemelum Nobile	Flowers	1.2.3.4	✗	✓	✓	✓	✓	Pre-anaesthetic, calms central nervous system, nervous asthma, neuralgia
Ylang Ylang	Cananga Odorata	Flowers	1.2.3.4	✗	✓	✓	✓	✗	Sexual exhaustion, relaxing and sedative, frigidity

Essential Oil Chart

Essential Oil Chart – Herbs

Essential Oil	Botanical name	Part of plant used	Method of use	Female massage Trimester 1	2	3	Male massage	Baby baths & massage	Main use in the family
Clary Sage	Salvia Sclarea	Leaves	Not Permitted	✗	✗	✗	✗	✗	Piles, nervous fatigue, aphrodisiac, can speed up stage 1 labour
Everlasting	Helichrysum Italicum	Flowers	1.2.3	✗	✗	✗	✗	✗	Bruises, ulcers, herpes, gingivitis, aphrodisiac?
Geranium	Pelagonium Asperum	Leaves	1.2.3.4	✗	✓	✓	✓	✗	Labour, fungal infections, skin problems, E.N.T. infections
Peppermint	Mentha Piperita	Leaves	1.2.3	✗	✗	✗	✗	✗	Nausea, heals open and infected wounds, anti-bacterial, anti-viral
Rock Rose	Cistus Ladaniferus	Branches/ Leaves	1.2.3	✗	✗	✗	✗	✗	Skin healing, stops bleeding, anti-viral
Geraniol Thyme	Thymus Vulgaris Geraniol	Leaves	1.2.3.4	✗	✗	✓	✓	✓	Labour, fungal infections, skin problems, E.N.T. infections

Essential Oil Chart - Trees

Essential Oil	Botanical name	Part of plant used	Method of use	Female massage Trimester 1	2	3	Male massage	Baby baths & massage	Main use in the family
Eucalyptus	Eucalyptus Radiata	Leaves	1.2.3.4	✗	✓	✓	✓	✓	Anti-viral against flu and colds etc.
Common Pine	Pinus Sylvestris	Needles	1.2.3.4	✗	✗	✓	✓	✗	Bronchitis, sinusitis, leg circulation, anti-fungal, exhaustion
Cypress	Cupressus Sempervirens	Branches	1.2.3.4	✗	Legs ✓	Legs ✓	✓	✗	Swollen legs/feet, piles, varicose veins, respiratory tract infections
Rosewood	Aniba Rosaeodora	Wood	1.2.3.4	✗	✓	✓	✓	✓	Anti-fungal, E.N.T. infection, exhaustion, anti-viral
Sandalwood	Santalum Album	Heartwood	1.2.3.4	✗	✓	✓	✓	✗	Lymph and vein decongestant, sedative, piles, aphrodisiac, certain lower back pains
Black Spruce	Picea Mariana	Needles	1.2.3.4	✗	✗	✓	✓	✗	Exhaustion, muscle pains, bronchitis, dry eczema
Tea Tree	Melaleuca Alternifolia	Leaves	1.2.3.4	✗	✓	✓	✓	✓	Use against ALL types of infections, exhaustion, helps leg circulation

88

Essential Oil Chart

Essential Oil Chart – Spices

Essential Oil	Botanical name	Part of plant used	Method of use	Female massage Trimester 1	2	3	Male massage	Baby baths & massage	Main use in the family
Cinnamon	Cinnamonum Verum	Leaves	1.2.3	✗	✗	✗	✓	✗	Anti-viral, male aphrodisiac, anti-fungal (Candida), for airborne infections
Clove	Eugenia Caryophyllus	Dry buds	4	✗	✗	✗	✗	✗	Excellent in use against airborne infections. Strengthens and tonifies the respiratory and nervous systems
Ginger	Zingiber Officinale	Rhizome	1.2.3	✗	✓	✗	✓	✗	Constipation, male aphrodisiac, muscular problems, helps digestion, anti-viral, nausea

KEY to method use

1 To fragrance a room

Do not use more than three different oils at a time, or you might both get overwhelmed. Keep to two, if you can. Put a lightbulb ring or tissue over heat source, and use one drop of each oil.

2. In the bath

Run your bath (not too hot) and add in three drops of your chosen oils. Swish it all around and get in. Predilute your essential oils in creamy milk or carrier oil if you have fair or sensitive skin.

3. In the shower

Put the plug in and drop 1-3 drops of your chosen oils onto the floor of the shower/bath. Turn on the hot water and adjust the temperature to suit you. Step in and breathe away.

4. Body massage

For a mum-to-be, use one drop of essential oil to every 5ml of carrier oil – in a 25ml bottle you can have 5 drops of essential oil, single or blended fragrance.

For the dad-to-be, you can go up to 3 drops to every 5ml or 15 drops to a 25ml bottle.

For a baby/child, use 1 drop to 10ml of carrier oil and two drops in 20ml. If an extra drop slips out, add 10ml of carrier oil to keep the strength correct.

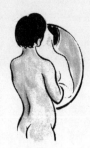

Index

Index